Medical Research and the Death Penalty

A DIALOGUE

JACK KEVORKIAN, M.D.

Medical Research and the Death Penalty

A DIALOGUE

VANTAGE PRESS NEW YORK WASHINGTON HOLLYWOOD

FIRST EDITION

Published by Vantage Press, Inc.
120 West 31st Street, New York 1, N. Y.

Manufactured in the United States of America

TO

the Hellenists of ancient Alexandria

Who evidently dared to do that which we scarcely

dare ponder

CONTENTS

MEDICAL RESEARCH AND THE DEATH PENALTY

A DIALOGUE

INTRODUCTION

You are to be more than a mere reader of this book. You are to be judge and jury, the instrument of practical logic. You may read these words earnestly, or frivolously; out of boredom, or because of a desire to think, weigh, and conclude. No matter what the motivation, it is hardly conceivable that you will be able to read them without arriving at a tentative or final decision regarding the central theme—as every good judge and jury should. Resolve, then, that this is your charge, and that it is you who will finally decide on the arguments and evidence to be exhibited in the incorruptible sanctuary of the court that is your soul.

The issue is a grave one, worthy of profound thought. It has been allowed to stagnate for over 2,000 years, and is fraught with the ideals our civilization embodies. It concerns law, medicine, sociology, and philosophy, and the overwhelming unknowns we call life and death. It is probably not new to some of you; but I feel certain that any acquaintance you might heretofore have had with it stems from an idea original with you or from private conversation with others. It deserves much more than the casual scrutiny presently accorded it. It deserves wide dissemination and concerted study.

You are no doubt wondering what issue could be so vitally important and yet have been neglected so long. A little over a year ago I presented a formal scientific paper before the American Society of Criminology at the annual meeting of the American Association for the Advancement of Science in Washington, D.C., in which I proposed that condemned men be allowed the choice of submitting to anesthesia and medical experimentation, as a form of execution, in lieu of conventional methods now prescribed by law.[1] Although the idea is essentially not a new one, I expected it to be controversial, but hardly as repugnant and shocking as the reception given it might indicate. All I wanted to do was to promote discussion.

But to my dismay discussion has been difficult, in fact impossible, to stimulate. The idea is publicly treated as a radical concept which will hurt or destroy the reputation of anyone connected with it. What little support there is has been expressed warily in public, yet freely to me in private. On the other hand, opposition has been open and vociferous; simply because opposing a "radical" idea is easily sanctioned and requires little courage. Many opponents, most of them well educated men of professional standing, have rejected the idea on emotional, irrelevant, or contradictory grounds. I have repeatedly challenged a few of them to debate before any audience of professional and lay people. Not one has answered the challenge. Not one has stated his reasons for refusing to answer. It is possible that they consider the issue too superficial to pursue further, although it is doubtful that any of them would admit such a total or even partial basis for his action.

That is the purpose of this book. My only recourse is to present such a debate to you as it would undoubtedly take place. As Protagonist I will face my opponent, the Antagonist; and in the following pages we will argue before you, as judge and jury. Each session will deal with a major aspect of the problem. The Antagonist has spoken to me already in the form of numerous newspaper and journal comments, personal letters, and private conversations. I know his stand well and will try to record it faithfully. Above all, objectivity is the aim. Arguments must be sound and irrefutable. They must be factual, or valid expressions of opinion based on fact. Emotion has no place in a court of justice and, therefore, no place in this debate.

Much, so very much, that is accessible and incredibly beneficial to human welfare hangs in the balance. This is a matter of supreme importance which transcends us and our time. Wisdom is the key. And with this one final request—that you judge sincerely within the limits of your innate wisdom—we enter your chambers and take our stands.

FIRST SESSION

The Problem

Antagonist: I must admit that this idea is quite new to me. As I understand it, it involves medical experimentation on men who are condemned to death. Is that correct?

Protagonist: Yes, that is entirely correct as far as you have gone. Let me reword the proposal so that you cannot fail to note all its implications. I propose that men condemned to death by due process of civil law during peacetime be allowed to submit, by their own free choice, to medical experimentation under surgical anesthesia, to be started at the set minute of execution and from which they will never awake. Is it clear now?

Antagonist: Indeed it is. But I would like to tell you at the outset that I am very strongly opposed to the idea of capital punishment. I feel that it has served no purpose whatsoever. There are cogent sociological and statistical studies which prove this point.[2]

Protagonist: What you say may or may not be true, and I appreciate your vigorous stand. However, please understand that this is not the basic issue at hand.

Antagonist: How can you say that? Unless I misunderstood, it was so defined in your opening statement.

Protagonist: Let me put it another way. I am sure that even if I wished to discuss the merits of the death penalty, my attempt could not begin to match the numerous books and treatises already dealing with the subject. It seems almost fruitless to me to delve into that controversy once again—one which has defied solution for many centuries and which is probably insoluble in terms of human existence. Both sides of the controversy are fraught with nothing but opinions, and . . .

Antagonist: Oh, but that is not so. I have already mentioned the statistical evidence which demonstrates that capital punishment has no deterrent effect upon the crime rate in this country. In fact the capital crime rate is lower in those states which have abolished the death penalty.[2]

Protagonist: Again, you may be right. I frankly admit that I do not know, but you must also understand that I do not care. Capital punishment is a legislated form of justice. That the death penalty exists is an inescapable reality. It is at this point that my proposal enters the discussion. The death penalty is the cause, my proposal its effect. Let me state it another way: wherever and whenever capital punishment is practiced, there is a far better way to implement it.

Antagonist: Now, what do you mean by "better way"?

Protagonist: That is something which will be clarified, but with your permission I should like to postpone it for the time being. The important point to be settled now is that the merits of capital punishment are of absolutely no concern to the problem under discussion.

Antagonist: Nevertheless, I am still unshakably opposed to the death penalty and equally opposed to anything which holds a promise of perpetuating it. Therefore, I am opposed to your proposal at the outset.

Protagonist: Let me try again, with a question. Does capital punishment exist in the United States today?

Antagonist: It does, of course.

Protagonist: Are men being executed?

Antagonist: Yes.

Protagonist: Disregarding the fact that you are opposed to any form of execution, do you feel that the methods now in vogue are desirable? In other words, would you be opposed to the introduction of a more humane way of execution?

Antagonist: My feeling about the death penalty makes it very distasteful to pursue this line of reasoning.

Protagonist: I appreciate your position and ask you to bear with me. Do you feel that executions as now carried out under civil law are being done in the best possible way?

Antagonist: What do you mean by the "best possible way"?

Protagonist: That is what I am trying to clarify. I mean the most efficient, humane, least torturous way.

Antagonist: That question deserves a great deal of thought. My first impression is that those states which make use of the gas chamber have come closest to the perfect way.

Protagonist: Then you feel that the gas chamber is the best possible way to execute a man.

Antagonist: No, I didn't say the best possible way. I said the best way now in practice. But on second thought I would say that it is the best possible way. I have read some articles on the effects of gas, and so far as I can determine it results in a very pleasant, smooth death.

Protagonist: Have you ever observed an execution in the gas chamber?

Antagonist: No, I haven't.

Protagonist: Have you ever inhaled cyanide gas?

Antagonist: No.

Protagonist: Have you ever seen an animal die of cyanide poisoning?

Antagonist: No.

Protagonist: Then upon what did you base your choice?

Antagonist: As I stated earlier, I based it on what I read and hear.

Protagonist: Well, then, if we assume that the gas chamber is the best way to carry out executions, what would you say of those states which use the electric chair?

Antagonist: My understanding is that the electric chair is not too bad, except for a momentary shock and perhaps a heating effect. I will admit that it might be a little less desirable than the gas chamber.

Protagonist: It follows from what you say that the electric chair is not the best means of carrying out executions. Do you agree?

Antagonist: Yes.

Protagonist: Then the actual implementation of the death penalty in many states leaves something to be desired?

Antagonist: You seem to be splitting hairs, but I guess I must agree with you on that point.

Protagonist: And what do you say of those states which use hanging?

Antagonist: I thought that form of execution disappeared long ago in the United States.

Protagonist: Let me assure you that it still exists in six states.

Antagonist: I will readily admit that hanging is a very undesirable way to carry out the death penalty. It is grotesque, to say the least.

Protagonist: What is your opinion of the firing squad?

Antagonist: Firing squad? Again you surprise me. I had no idea that such an archaic method was still in use.

Protagonist: One state offers the condemned a choice between the firing squad and hanging. Don't you agree that that is not an enviable position to be in?

Antagonist: Most certainly. I would classify the former as perhaps a little more pleasant. However, some people are of the opinion that hanging itself, contrary to all external appearances, is a rapid and not too unpleasant way to die.

Protagonist: Of all these methods; gas chamber, electrocution, hanging, firing squad, and, to add a fifth, the guillotine, which would you choose if you were a condemned man?

Antagonist: If I had to choose among the five alternatives, I believe I would prefer the gas chamber.

Protagonist: How would you list your choices, progressing from the most desirable to the most abhorrent?

Antagonist: The most desirable for me would be the gas chamber, second electrocution, then the firing squad, guillotine, and hanging. The last three are difficult to separate preferentially because they are all so undesirable.

Protagonist: Your choices correspond to those of others to whom I have posed the same question. Now let me ask you point-blank: Do you believe that there is a better way to die than in the gas chamber?

Antagonist: It is hard to imagine offhand, but I suppose there is a better way.

Protagonist: That is what I wanted to hear from you, regarding the possibility of the best form of execution.

Antagonist: However, if there is such a way, I am not acquainted with it.

Protagonist: Have you ever been under anesthesia in a hospital?

Antagonist: Yes. I once had ether for a relatively minor operation.

Protagonist: Was it unpleasant?

Antagonist: Well, it wasn't the most exhilarating experience in the world. There was a disagreeable burning effect in my throat.

Protagonist: Have you ever been under influence of sodium pentothal?

Antagonist: What is that?

Protagonist: It is a liquid drug of the barbiturate class used to produce very pleasant sleep by slow injection into a vein. Then ether and other conventional gases are used to maintain the anesthetic state during surgery. There are absolutely no adverse effects.

Antagonist: Because I have never had the drug, it is difficult for me to form an opinion regarding its effects.

Protagonist: Do you think that death due to an overdose of sleeping pills would be horrible to experience?

Antagonist: No, I think that is one of the easiest ways to die.

Protagonist: Do you feel that such a death is more pleasant than that caused with cyanide gas?

Antagonist: I would guess that they were about the same.

Protagonist: That is probably not true. I have seen a solution of cyanide, poured into the stomach of a rabbit through a tube, kill the animal in a matter of minutes, with violent terminal convulsions. It was not in the least pleasant to the observers. And the effect of cyanide on a living body is always the same whether the body gets it by drinking a solution or by breathing the gas.

Antagonist: I had no idea that cyanide caused convulsions. I thought it merely produced a pleasant sleep, a sort of drowsiness that gradually overtook a person.

Protagonist: Your description leads me to conclude that insofar as you know, its effect is identical to an overdose of sleeping pills. If you were given the choice of dying by cyanide or by sleeping pills, which would you take?

Antagonist: I believe I would prefer the sleeping pills.

Protagonist: Which is tantamount to choosing death under pentothal anesthesia. That is exactly what I advocate through my proposal—a new and better method of execution. Death for the condemned would amount to a very rapid induction of sleep from which he would never awake. And the instant of induction of that sleep would correspond exactly with the instant set for throwing the switch or dropping the gas pellets.

Antagonist: It seems to me that anesthetic execution offers so small a gain over the gas chamber that it's hardly worth discussing, much less legislating, as a new form of destroying the condemned.

Protagonist: Please do not judge the entire proposal on this single facet. I am not simply dabbling with the concept of the death penalty. A new form of execution is only one constituent of a complex which embodies so many enormous advantages that to disparage it because of one aspect borders on the ridiculous. We must first establish this fact: namely, that there *is* a better form of execution and that it involves induction of surgical anesthesia with intravenous sodium pentothal. This point alone may not convince anyone of the merit of the entire proposal, but in conjunction with the others to follow it should be more than enough to sway any reasonable man.

Antagonist: That remains to be seen. I still feel that anesthesia offers little subjective advantage over the other methods high on my list.

Protagonist: You make an erroneous assumption which, I am sorry to say, is too easily made. What we observe objectively in the death of another can hardly be equated with what the person experiences subjectively. If a man dies under cyanide gas without convulsing, we might infer that his death was serene and pleasant. But we fail to note that cyanide kills by choking, by cutting off the supply of oxygen to the energy centers of his body's cells. This amounts to cutting off his air. Now it seems to me that to suffocate is not a pleasant way to die. The same is true of hanging. When the trap door is sprung and the body falls rapidly, the neck is quickly broken. It is consequently assumed that the man dies quickly and therefore, easily. But how can we be so sure that the man himself is not thrown into the most horrible chaos? For the cervical spine is broken and the spinal cord severed. We can never be sure of what is passing through the victim's mind—so-called "spinal shock" notwithstanding.

So far as electrocution is concerned, is it not rational to assume that the passage of a high-voltage charge through a known electrical organ such as the brain might temporarily disrupt normal physiology in a manner capable of engendering an indescribably terrifying state of consciousness? Furthermore, electrical charges do not always kill a man instantaneously; for their lethal effect depends more on frequency of current than on magnitude of voltage. Many of us have heard of instances in which more than one attempt was necessary to stop finally the heart of a condemned man. Repeated electrical shocks create heat. And to experience this in addition to the actual shocking effect of high-voltage charges cannot be construed as a pleasant way to die. When the head is lopped off by the guillotine or the heart ripped out by bullets, who can say what passes through the victim's mind? What appears to us as a pleasant death, because apparently instantaneous, may be extremely torturous.

Antagonist: All this is very interesting. Do you mean that when a man is dying in a tranquil fashion, his death may not, for himself, be tranquil in a mental or psychic sense?

Protagonist: That is exactly what I mean. Do you personally know of any instance in which a person underwent the process of execution as now practiced and survived to tell about it?

Antagonist: I do not.

Protagonist: On the other hand, do you personally know of anyone who submitted to pentothal induction for anesthesia prior to surgery and survived to tell about it?

Antagonist: I know of people who were anesthetized, but I am not sure if pentothal was used.

Protagonist: Well, I can take you to any hospital in the country and introduce you to many such patients and have them tell you of the experience. Do you think that they would characterize it as unpleasant?

Antagonist: They would probably say that it was not very unpleasant.

Protagonist: Now perhaps you have grasped the point I wish to make. On the one hand we have literally thousands of examples of sleep characterized as pleasant by the subjects themselves. On the other hand, we have not one such direct verification by any victim of the other methods producing unconsciousness and eventual death. All I am advocating is that we substitute a procedure which we *know* to be tolerable for one which we *surmise* may be tolerable.

Antagonist: I don't doubt your logic, but I still think you are splitting hairs.

Protagonist: Then I have settled the point satisfactorily. I am proposing a new method of execution known to be pleasant. Therefore, I am not trying to introduce a disadvantageous variable into the controversy over capital punishment. If you or anyone else doubts the subjective serenity of anesthetic death as compared with conventional execution, you are in fact saying that the thousands of patients undergoing surgery risk a death subjectively more distasteful than that inflicted under the death penalty. Will you admit to such a stand?

Antagonist: It would be difficult to justify such a viewpoint.

Protagonist: Agreed, then, that anesthesia offers the most desirable way of ending the life of a condemned man.

Antagonist: Nevertheless I am still strongly opposed to the practice of capital punishment, and introducing a better way of carrying it out does not by any means make the concept acceptable to me.

Protagonist: We will touch upon this point again, but for now I am satisfied if we have established the fact that the method of execution embodied in my proposal is advantageous, and that this advantage will be magnified as the ramifications of this complex problem unfold.

Antagonist: Now that you mention ramifications, I would like to know exactly what they are. Specifically how do you propose to carry out this plan?

SECOND SESSION

The Plan

Protagonist: The plan itself is simple enough in theory, and I am sure that it could be made almost equally simple in practice. Once a person has been condemned to death, he will be informed at the time of sentencing that he may die either by the method prescribed by law in that state, or by submitting to anesthesia, from which he will never awaken, for the purpose of allowing medical experimentation.

Antagonist: You mean, then, that the judge will inform the condemned of this choice when sentence is passed?

Protagonist: Exactly. I believe I can explain the more detailed mechanisms of the plan by using a hypothetical example. Let us assume that a man of approximately 30 is found guilty of murder in the first degree in a state where executions involve hanging.

Antagonist: Well, now, you have picked a mode of execution which is very distasteful, and I feel certain that a condemned man would prefer your advocated alternative merely to avoid a horrible death.

Protagonist: This point concerning the relative degrees of pleasantness of the various modes of death has not been satisfactorily clarified, and we will return to that later. Nevertheless your criticism is valid. I will change hanging to the gas chamber in my example. Is that acceptable to you?

Antagonist: That is acceptable. It helps restore balance to your example.

Protagonist: Very well. Let us assume that the condemned killer faces a judge who sentences him to death in the gas chamber. The judge at that time informs the man that he may choose to die instead under anesthesia for the purpose of medical research; that anesthesia will be induced by painless intravenous injection of a sleeping drug; that while he is under anesthesia, competent researchers will carry out studies on his living body; and that at the end of the experiments, which may last for hours or for weeks, death will be brought about by an overdose of the anesthetic agent.

Antagonist: I would like to interrupt at this point to raise the question of death brought about by experimentation. Would that possibility be explained also?

Protagonist: That's a good point. If death were to occur accidentally while the experiment was in progress, the sentence of the court would have been carried out. The man would never regain consciousness, and for him death would correspond to the actual instant of induction of sleep—or when the cyanide pellets would have been dropped into the acid. If the condemned's living body were to endure the experiment successfully, ultimate death could easily be brought about by an overdose of anesthetic. Can you detect any barbarity in what I have just outlined?

Antagonist: I really cannot, although the idea of being experimented upon for days does not strike my fancy.

Protagonist: But you must admit that, being under total anesthesia, you would in every practical sense be dead.

Antagonist: Yes, what you say is true, although it is esthetically disagreeable to me.

Protagonist: Good, then I will continue. The man is taken to the death house to await execution. While there, he is allowed to contemplate the choice facing him. He is not asked for a decision until one week prior to the set date. Let us assume that execution has been set for one full year after the day of condemnation. The man thus has a year for deliberation and consultation with legal and medical authorities, in order to insure that he clearly understands his predicament. Consultation will be given as freely and compassionately as possible.

One week prior to the set date of execution he is approached by special representatives of the medical and legal professions and asked for a tentative decision. If, at this time, the condemned chooses to die under the conditions of my plan, the initial steps are now taken to set up the experiment, which, of necessity, will have to be located at a nearby research center sufficiently well equipped and staffed to do justice to the studies planned. Two days are allowed for the condemned to reverse his decision. If he does so, all plans for experimentation are immediately halted and the man is doomed to execution in the gas chamber.

However, if he sticks to his tentative decision, all preparations go into high gear. I would be inclined to limit the man to only one reversal of his tentative decision, in order to minimize the purposeless and wasteful vacillation of a mind which may perhaps be overly burdened or just plain malicious.

Antagonist: What if the condemned man is not perfectly sure of his choice? What if his external appearance and behavior seemed to belie what he says?

Protagonist: All plans for experimentation will be dropped without hesitation if, in the opinion of those authorities present, the condemned appears to be uncertain or fearful. Only those men who are absolutely sure that my plan offers them the best way to die will be candidates for it.

Antagonist: I see. I heartily endorse the stringent conditions involved. Please continue.

Protagonist: At that crucial time, when the man has less than a week to live, his entire case is submitted to the supreme court of the state concerned for a final, thorough review. It might even be submitted to the Supreme Court of the United States which should perhaps have the ultimate adjudication in this undeniably grave matter. The man's conviction and sentence must be upheld, and the conditions surrounding his final choice must pass thorough scrutiny at this high level. If all is found to be in order, then the projected plan will be implemented. However, any doubt about the validity of any aspect of the circumstances leading to this point will be grounds for complete termination of further preparations or for postponement pending clarification of the sources of such doubt.

Antagonist: That is certainly fair enough, and I suppose we now assume that the high court in your hypothetical example has given the green light for continuation of execution as planned.

Protagonist: Yes. On the day of execution the condemned man is transported under heavy guard and physical restraints to the institute at which the study is to be carried out. In a clean, hospital-like atmosphere he is put to sleep at the exact second prescribed for his execution. For all practical purposes he is now quite dead. His condition corresponds exactly to the state of clinical death from which patients may occasionally be resuscitated by cardiac massage. I call it *clinical death;* a term meaning that part of non-existence which is especially characterized by the possibility of being resuscitated. A man on an operating table undergoing execution under anesthesia could be resuscitated, although he is clinically dead.

Antagonist: In other words, you are comparing clinical death with coma, as seen in certain accident victims or patients having brain tumors, for example?

Protagonist: Correct. For me there is absolutely no subjective difference between dreamless sleep, deep coma, any kind of unconsciousness, and clinical death in which heartbeat, respiration, pulse, and blood pressure are undetectable.

Antagonist: That is a large order for me to swallow. Although our definitions do not coincide very well, I will admit that the subjective states in all these instances would probably be about the same.

Protagonist: Our concepts seem to coincide pretty well, however. Recent progress in clinical practice has made the phenomenon of death difficult to define; indeed impossible. Nobody can really define that nebulous and fleeting span in which revocable life ends and the one-way road to extinction begins. Earlier, death was simply defined as the cessation beyond recall of indispensable physiological processes of the intact organism; when all vital signs were no longer detectable, and therefore assumed to be absent, the man was pronounced dead. But today we know very well that a man in such a state can be resuscitated, even to a fully conscious and apparently normal life in some instances.

Antagonist: I don't believe we need carry this discussion any further. Let me just acknowledge again that subjectively unconsciousness, coma and clinical death probably amount to the same thing.

Protagonist: That acknowledgement is sufficient for my purposes. So we now have the condemned man on the operating table under pentothal anesthesia, and for practical purposes, dead. The experimentation itself can begin in ten to fifteen minutes, when other anesthetic agents, such as ether, nitrous oxide, or cyclopropane, have been used to reach and maintain the desired level of anesthesia. These agents are in common use in hospitals and are known to be tolerated with no adverse subjective effects.

Antagonist: I would like to interrupt. Just who would be allowed to witness these proceedings? Only the medical team?

Protagonist: No, I would hesitate to limit attendance to just these scientists. It seems reasonable that the audience include lawyers, judges, and perhaps theologians and philosophers. This would ensure that the entire undertaking would be in sincere good taste, above the slightest reproach, and aimed at the most noble ends.

Antagonist: I can hardly find fault with such stipulations. But let's go on. The man is now undergoing experimentation. How long should this reasonably go on?

Protagonist: We cannot be certain of the length of time which any given project might take. Some experiments may last no longer than a few hours. Others will of necessity stretch out for days or even weeks.

Antagonist: Weeks! This is barbarous!

Protagonist: May I remind you of what we have already agreed concerning subjective experiences under anesthesia? No matter how long this condition is maintained, so long as it is strictly controlled the subject can never be aware of existence.

Antagonist: Agreed. But I am now raising an esthetic objection, which seriously detracts from the desirability of your plan, to say the least.

Protagonist: There is some knowledge regarding human health and illness which cannot be acquired in any other way than by direct experimentation upon living human subjects, and some of these experiments must be protracted.

Antagonist: Could you cite a few pertinent examples?

Protagonist: I would be glad to. But since a subsequent session will be devoted entirely to medical aspects of the plan, may I defer my answer?

Antagonist: Certainly. I'll make a mental note of that. It should be an interesting session.

Protagonist: Because of your understandable concern about possible subjective experiences, let me state that I believe that anesthesia should be controlled day and night by a team of anesthesiologists—at the very least by two such specialists. Would that not ensure a continual state of "death" for the condemned?

Antagonist: It would, indeed.

Protagonist: If, as I stated before, experimentation does not cause the subject's irreversible death, that can be induced at the end of the experiment by an overdose of the anesthetic agent. I can think of no calmer way to die.

Antagonist: What happens when the experiment is thus concluded?

Protagonist: At that point conventional legal machinery for the disposition of the body is put into motion. That aspect requires no discussion.

Antagonist: I have two questions which are very important. First, what type of medical study would be carried out and who would perform it; and, secondly, how would the entire plan be administered, that is, through what organization could it be most smoothly implemented?

Protagonist: Those are very basic questions, and please do not forget that this outline is strictly hypothetical. However, in answer to your questions, it would seem to me advisable to have proposed experiments from all over the civilized world, devised especially to take advantage of these sacrificial occasions, funneled into a central coordinating agency; perhaps most logically one within the framework of the United Nations. That is to say that scientists of any nation who feel that they have experiments capable of giving mankind valuable information about the functioning of the human organism, information obtainable from no other source than the living human body, could outline their plans in detail and submit them to the agency for evaluation. The agency itself should consist of members of the medical and allied professions, all of whom are of national or international repute and have demonstrated exceptional competence. Their number is not important; their integrity, however, must be unquestioned. This international body would assess the relative merits of submitted plans, with the prime objective of selecting those plans which held greatest promise of benefiting mankind. But immediate benefit itself would not be the chief aim in some instances. Some studies would be aimed at revealing the great principles underlying normal physiology and at helping us in the gigantic struggle to understand what human life really means. Once a plan had been selected, its authors would be alerted for transportation to that nation which had available a man who had chosen this method of execution.

Antagonist: How would the agency be made aware of these opportunities?

Protagonist: I neglected to mention that the same agency would automatically be notified by all civilized nations of impending executions within their borders, and of the tentative dates of these executions. If the condemned man was deemed suitable for the experiment then the chosen team would be transported to the nation of execution. If the equipment in that nation was inadequate, the team could bring along its own. These are all minor details which are easily eradicable, and which tend to obscure the more basic issues.

Antagonist: I would not be inclined to dispose of the details so lightly. Money is always an important consideration, and isn't this idea of transporting teams and equipment all over the world expensive? And chaotic?

Protagonist: On the surface it would appear to be. May I again suggest that we reserve this point, too, for a later session? Instead let me interject this one thought: do you think that the prospect of a little chaos should deter a scientist from going to any lengths to probe the profound secrets of human life, death, and disease? The prospect of chaos does not deter me, for the road to the solution of these enigmas will be far more chaotic than any plan man can conceive. And the prospect of spending large sums of money while on that road is the last consideration that should enter the scientist's mind. We Americans today are the wealthiest nation on earth, and are supporting research to the tune of many millions of dollars annually. A few profound experiments on condemned men would make many animal and "test tube" projects now in progress completely superfluous. Thus the cost in some fields of research would not only not be increased, but would actually be reduced.

Antagonist: Well, then, it seems that I have most of the details I requested at the start of this session. It is possible, according to your plan, for an experimental project originating in the mind of a Russian researcher to be carried out in the state of Texas. Or an Australian may work in Guatemala.

Protagonist: That is absolutely correct.

Antagonist: But isn't all this a little absurd? Ideally your plan is rather nice. But that isn't the way the world runs, is it?

Protagonist: You're right, but now let's become practical. You have admitted that ideally my position is sound. It may not be the best one in a practical sense, but I am sure that it is at least feasible in the United States. We pride ourselves on being the world's leader in enlightenment. Ours is a wealthy nation, and men are being executed in many of our states every year. I am sure that the plan is practicable within *our* borders. If a man is condemned in one state, a plan devised by a scientist in any other state could easily be carried out in that state, could it not?

Antagonist: Yes, I see your point. In other words, rather than dealing with the world, you are now reverting to the states of our nation which practice capital punishment.

Protagonist: Yes. Instead of the United Nations administering the plan, we could entrust it to the Supreme Court, which would work through the highest courts of the states involved. Is the plan still only theoretically correct, or has it now assumed the aura of practical feasibility which a materialistic age so steadfastly demands? We might thereby set an example for the world to follow.

Antagonist: I will admit that it has become somewhat more practical. Nevertheless I think the obstacles, even in our nation, are enormous, even insurmountable at present.

Protagonist: I see it that way, too. The plan offers an unusual change, and change is never lightly accepted. It is slow in coming about, but it always evolves where there is a *will* to see it evolve. What is important is that the will be there.

Antagonist: Perhaps time will be kind to your proposal. In the meantime I grant that it has theoretical merit and practical possibilities. I can go no further than that.

Protagonist: Fair enough. To say that such a plan could not be implemented in the United States would be tantamount to admitting that we either are incapable of doing so or do not desire to do so. There is no other alternative. I personally feel that we *are* capable of administering such a plan; at least I would reserve admission of incapability until after a fair trial. If, then, we do not institute a trial run during the course of the next few decades, I will be forced to conclude that we do not desire it.

Antagonist: What you are saying, then, is simply that if such a plan is never put into effect, it reflects derogatorily on the group rejecting it without trial. Isn't that a rather harsh judgment to make?

Protagonist: Yes, but justifiably so. Let me ask you point-blank: Is the plan practicable in the United States?

Antagonist: Yes, it is.

Protagonist: Assuming that the plan is a progressive step, then, if it is not implemented in a nation capable of doing so, is that not a disparagement of that nation?

Antagonist: Yes, under the conditions stated. But your assumption is enormous, and I am not willing to grant it.

Protagonist: I did not ask for concurrence with my assumption. I merely wanted to know your reaction *assuming* that one fact. Would it then not be disparaging?

Antagonist: Yes, making that one great assumption, it would. But it is definitely up to you to show that the plan would indeed benefit mankind to an extent which would outweigh its distasteful aspects; that it would be a progressive step in the evolution of our civilization.

Protagonist: That is the explicit purpose of this debate. We have established a fundamental point. The most pressing question to be answered is whether or not the plan is a progressive or retrogressive step, and that will have been done in the course of these sessions. The problem is far too great to be solved in a single session. It may be presumptuous of me even to think that it can be done at all, but I believe it can.

Antagonist: It *is* a challenging question, but I am convinced of my ability to show you that your plan is really an evil one. At any rate, let us backtrack from these abstractions to the abject position of the condemned man himself. As I understand this session, everything really hinges on him. I am not so sure that many condemned persons would choose your proposed method.

Protagonist: That may or may not be correct. I hope I have satisfactorily clarified for you the tentative mechanism of my plan. Now let's consider how the condemned man himself might fit into the workings of that mechanism. You are right when you say that he is a key figure, for everything revolves around his decision.

THIRD SESSION

The Condemned

Antagonist: What is your opinion regarding the enormous burden which would be placed upon the condemned facing such a decision?

Protagonist: The question is certainly fair enough, and will serve admirably to get this session off to a good start. As I see it, the plan can hardly be disadvantageous to a condemned man. The choice in the matter is his entirely.

Antagonist: I don't think you grasp the meaning of my question. Don't you feel that such a grave decision would weigh heavily upon the man's sense of well-being?

Protagonist: That's a valid opinion, and I don't doubt that on the surface such a decision would indeed trouble the man. But do not forget that it opens up an avenue of escape from the horrible fate awaiting him, a fate not pleasant to anticipate. Now we offer him instead a far more pleasant death, both from the physical and psychical standpoints; and, in addition, give him the opportunity to gain a sense of utility in dying.

Antagonist: It is easy to overlook the fact that this man's mind is full of chaotic and despondent thoughts. When another variable is introduced it appears, at first glance, to hold out promise of alleviating the victim's burden. But no matter what the variable promises in the way of a humane death it will operate as just one more unpredictable variable taxing the condemned man's already overburdened psychic reserve. In my opinion, this plan can do no good which would justify the inevitably resulting damage. Apparently condemned men soon resign themselves to their fate, and I would rather leave our present system with its deficiencies intact than take the immense risk you advocate.

Protagonist: It is difficult to come to any sort of conclusion about the subjective reactions you posit. I can offer some insight into a possible solution by suggesting that you imagine yourself as a condemned man. Would you prefer to know that you will go to the gas chamber at a set time, or instead to have the privilege of choosing between that alternative and death under anesthesia amounting to nothing more than undergoing surgery in a hospital?

Antagonist: I doubt whether I'd prefer to have the choice. There is not much appeal in the prospect of submitting to anesthesia and knowing that one may be vivisected while asleep. I realize I have already admitted that one would be unconscious of the proceedings. Nevertheless, there is something in human nature, some intangible tendency, which causes most men to shy away from anything ostensibly barbaric to other observers. Furthermore, I said earlier that the gas chamber is probably not really an unpleasant death; and anesthesia can in all likelihood offer little more as a tolerable lethal agent.

Protagonist: It is dismaying to have to revert constantly to points that we had considered settled. Many people undergo surgery with anesthesia every day and recover without apparent ill effects. However, we as observers have no way of determining the subjective experiences of a man who has suffered poisoning with cyanide to the extent of total unconsciousness. So far as I know, nobody has recovered from such a state to tell about it.

Antagonist: Still, on the basis of what we can infer from observation, it seems to me that anesthetic and cyanide deaths are equally smooth.

Protagonist: Let me ask another question: would you prefer

to die in the electric chair, or by hanging rather than under anesthesia?

Antagonist: If you insist on such grotesque alternatives, I would be inclined to choose anesthesia.

Protagonist: Well—you now admit, in a roundabout way, that you would rather have a choice if you were a condemned man.

Antagonist: I didn't say that.

Protagonist: But you definitely implied it by admitting that you would prefer anesthesia to hanging.

Antagonist: Yes, in that instance I would rather have the choice.

Protagonist: Then the plan would be worthwhile, if for no other reason than to give men now faced with death by hanging, or the electric chair, a choice.

Antagonist: I cannot go along with that entirely. You are asking me to agree that the plan should be put into effect, and I have told you that I am opposed to that.

Protagonist: Your stand is paradoxical. If you yourself would rather be faced with a choice were you condemned, yet refuse to grant it to others now actually in that predicament, are you not being somewhat hypocritical?

Antagonist: Don't forget that I am opposed to anything which would help foster the concept of capital punishment, and I . . .

Protagonist: Please excuse the interruption. I do not want to get embroiled in a fruitless discussion on the merits of the death penalty. I believe it is the idea of experimentation that is so repulsive to you. If that were not involved, would you agree that as long as capital punishment is in effect all currently used methods of execution should be discarded in favor of anesthesia?

Antagonist: When you state it in those terms it would be difficult for anyone not to agree.

Protagonist: Then in that respect my plan is a definite improvement. But I refuse to divorce experimentation from anesthesia. It is not subjectively intolerable, nor is it barbaric, and it will, contrary to your fears, make the plan unimaginably more beneficial. Of course, as you pointed out earlier, that is for me to prove. To get back to our hypothetical situation, your desire to have a choice between hanging and anesthesia even *with* experimentation seems to have settled our previous point of contention —that the psychologically burdened mind of a condemned man would not be further taxed if my choice were offered him.

Antagonist: I'm afraid my own admission damns me. I agree.

Protagonist: There is another even more serious circumstance which is definitely not hypothetical and which should further strengthen my argument. Tell me, have innocent men been executed?

Antagonist: According to what I have heard, they have. After all, we humans are fallible.

Protagonist: Very well. Now, if an innocent man is doomed to die, wouldn't he feel just a little bit better about it if he had the choice my plan would offer him?

Antagonist: I doubt that anything could allay the man's just anger, or despair. Are you trying to justify your plan by using it to rationalize the inexcusable killing of innocent men?

Protagonist: Not at all. No one can deny the tragedy involved in executing innocent men. But let's say that you were such a man. Wouldn't it make some difference to you how you were to die?

Antagonist: I suppose that I might wish at least to have an easy, tolerable death.

Protagonist: Certainly, that would be the more normal reaction. Otherwise you would be admitting that your sense of outrage had so clouded all of your positive values as to lead you to a blind and reckless expression of contempt. What kind of memory would you wish to leave with your family: that of an unjustly condemned man who was gassed, or one who died to give all of us knowledge and hope?

Antagonist: The latter, to be sure. But let me emphasize that just because innocent men have been executed I, and many other abolitionists, are doubly certain that the death penalty must be written off the books.

Protagonist: But remember that innocent or not, the man must by law die. Can you deny that as things now stand my plan would lighten the burden, the unimaginable mental anguish, of an innocent but doomed man?

Antagonist: No, I cannot.

Protagonist: There is still another consideration, although it is hardly applicable in our country. We read of revolutions and counterrevolutions in various nations of the world. After each upheaval there is usually a bloodbath of executions.

Antagonist: I know what you mean. A notorious one took place recently in Iraq.

Protagonist: And several high-ranking officials of the fallen regime were promptly tried and executed. The most recent episode occurred in Cuba, and you undoubtedly were incensed, as were all rational men, on reading of the mass executions by firing squad after mock trials in a carnival atmosphere.

Antagonist: The whole civilized world was appalled. But what does this have to do with the topic under discussion?

Protagonist: Just this: many of the victims of these post-revolution condemnations were men of standing, education, and some integrity. They simply had the misfortune to be on the losing side. They were condemned for political reasons. If they are not criminals in the conventional sense, why should they be forced to die like criminals? If they must die, don't you think my proposed choice would somewhat lighten their yoke and, at the same time, be more in line with their personal ideals as well as with those of society?

Antagonist: I do. But I also think you have gone somewhat far afield, and I suggest we return to the central theme of this session.

Protagonist: Can you anticipate any other disadvantages as far as the condemned man is concerned?

Antagonist: I cannot. But if he doesn't really understand what is to be done with his body should he agree to submit himself?

Protagonist: I have outlined that already. Official representatives of the medical and legal professions will always be available to answer his questions.

Antagonist: What will the condemned's family have to say about all this?

Protagonist: Absolutely nothing as far as I know. Once a man is condemned, his life is no longer his own, and much less so his family's. It belongs to the state. The relationship of the family to my plan will be touched upon later in more detail.

Antagonist: One more point. Don't you think that all these negotiations will lead to absurd delays and a waste of time and effort?

Protagonist: Not at all. As I stated in the last session, the man is approached one week prior to the date set for execution and asked for a decision. He can reverse his decision only once within the following two days. The man who wavers will not be considered a suitable candidate and will be executed in the conventional manner.

Antagonist: Won't this plan kill any "eleventh hour" chances of stay of execution or commutation of sentence? After all, there have been instances of executions only hours before the discovery of ameliorating or exonerating evidence.

Protagonist: You have brought up a point which adds substantial support to my proposal. You will remember that it called for induction of anesthesia at the set minute of execution. In other words anesthesia would never shorten the man's conscious life. What is of even greater importance, it would always *lengthen* the period of his vitality. Instead of dying when the switch was thrown, under anesthesia the man's body would be maintained in a perfectly resuscitable state for hours and sometimes days. If the experiment was not excessively mutilating or of such a nature as to be irreversibly injurious to health, the subject could conceivably be revived if evidence of innocence was uncovered. Now, instead of ruining "eleventh hour" chances of commutation, my plan would create "thirteenth" and even "fourteenth hour" chances. I feel that there are men now dead who today would be alive and free had my plan been in practice. This may seem like sentimentality, but if you or a loved one were concerned, it would literally mean the world.

Antagonist: It's very hard for me to muster arguments against these considerations. One final point—wouldn't the transfer of the prisoner to the site of research create an added chance of escape?

Protagonist: It might, yes. However, if this plan were in effect and an appreciable number of men were condemned in any given state each year, it might be advisable to construct special research-facilities at the prison. This would eliminate possibilities of escape.

Antagonist: But that would undoubtedly cost an excessive amount of money. It wouldn't be very practicable.

Protagonist: It would cost a lot of money, but medical research—research of any kind—is always expensive. Throughout history, as a rule, only prosperous, wealthy nations have been able to afford the luxury of research. If it proved too expensive, the only alternative would be to transport the man to an institute under heavy guard and restraints. If this, too, was not feasible, then perhaps the man could be moved while under deep anesthesia induced at the prison. Escape would then be out of the question. These are details that have no real bearing on the problem. Once the plan is instituted, they can all be easily resolved.

Antagonist: But it is difficult to grasp the full importance of your principles without delving into these details. They add color and body, they put a little meat on the bones, so to speak.

Protagonist: Yes, they do. I also find it refreshing to detour from time to time, but the framework should always stand out. Do you have any further questions?

Antagonist: I do not at this time. It seems to me that the most important points have been raised and elucidated. Some of them could perhaps have been pursued in more detail, but for our immediate purposes I think they have been sufficiently well covered.

FOURTH SESSION

The Laws

Antagonist: What's next on the agenda?

Protagonist: In this session I would like to discuss how the proposal might affect the laws governing executions. Specifically, I should like to determine whether or not it would be beneficial to the legal profession.

Antagonist: In this respect I can think of one big objection to the proposal. Would it not involve serious tampering with the *formality* of these laws? After all, the time and manner of executions are specifically prescribed by law in order to maintain the objectivity of justice, which is a man-made thing and easily corrupted. I feel that if these stipulations were altered, the possibility of corruption would be proportionately greater.

Protagonist: But just how radical *is* the tampering I propose? It amounts to nothing more than prescribing a new method of execution. Instead of the gallows, the gas chamber, or the electric chair, I merely advocate that the condemned be put to death with anesthesia. I can see therein no real meddling with the fundamental formality of the laws. The laws dictate execution for commission of a capital crime. Any convicted man is therefore a candidate for execution. The next legal step is the prescription of the manner of execution, which in most states is either gas or electrocution. I propose that these be supplemented by anesthetization. In reality they should be totally abolished in favor of anesthesia, but I do not advocate that extreme. To your way of thinking does that amount to dangerous tampering?

Antagonist: It does not, but the first step in any kind of conceptual change very often results in radical changes totally out of line with the original intentions. I would therefore oppose changes of any sort no matter how insignificant they might seem at their inception.

Protagonist: Please bear in mind that I am not proposing this change in order to achieve an insignificant and superficial end. The end in view is enormous and, to my mind, justifies the action. It would be up to us to guard against the introduction of radical measures.

Antagonist: Where will all this conjecture get us? You are ready to introduce what you describe as a benign step and then draw the line on further tampering. Some people would consider that initial step radical. To others, additional measures might still be insignificant and benign. Who is to say when and where the lines are to be drawn?

You maintain that the end in view is enormous, and I agree. But I hold the opinion that human nature is incapable of tampering without exceeding acceptable limits. Therefore, I would be inclined to reject the idea of any tampering with the laws as they now stand.

Protagonist: Earlier you stated that you are against capital punishment. Accordingly, you must feel that the practice should be abolished entirely. In my opinion that is a greater degree of tampering than any change I have proposed.

Antagonist: It's difficult to answer that objection satisfactorily. In order to keep a logical stand, I must insist that the present laws not change.

Protagonist: You seem to be in the dilemma of wanting to maintain current laws in order to preserve the integrity of your argument against my proposal, while this insistence belies your own fundamental belief that capital punishment is a bad thing and should be abolished. No such dilemma exists for me. I recognize the changeable character of human nature and of the human laws which emanate from it. I know that capital punishment is not a perfect form of meting out justice and that it will change eventually. The methods of its execution are crude and imperfect, and they will also change. Such a change is what I propose. My outlook is based on change: that change for the better which we call progress.

Antagonist: But my so-called dilemma is solvable. I did not make the laws regarding capital punishment. Because I know that it is evil, were I a legislator, I would have opposed its institution. And I am now opposed to its practice. If I advocate changing the law, I want to change it so that it corresponds to my basic philosophy. Where is the contradiction?

Protagonist: I believe we are missing an important distinction. What you propose is that a law be dropped from the statute books entirely. I advocate enactment of a new law to supplement those already in existence. Now, what we must decide is whether or not these amount to tampering with the *formality* of the legal system. If so, then every new law and every act of repeal is just as dangerous a form of tampering as what I suggest. Or would tampering be judged depending on the degree of the projected statutory change?

Antagonist: It is difficult to define tampering in those terms. Perhaps it would be better to say that tampering amounts to altering the mechanism whereby laws reach the statute books.

Protagonist: But that, too, simply involves adding and subtracting laws. The Constitution of the United States is a giant body of laws which define the mechanism of other laws. It seems that the dilemma affects us both, and results from the lack of a common definition.

Antagonist: You mean that it would be senseless to proceed further on this point?

Protagonist: Yes. You would so change the law as to abolish

capital punishment. Would the aim in view justify the change?

Antagonist: Yes.

Protagonist: And would the change amount to tampering with the *formality* of the law?

Antagonist: Hardly.

Protagonist: So, too, when I advocate this new form of execution. Neither of us considers himself to be tampering simply because the aim of his action is justification enough. Because our aims do not coincide, we can come to no common understanding. Despite this, will you grant that my proposal amounts to no more tampering with the formality of the law than that change which you advocate?

Antagonist: That seems fair enough, although it is obvious that any conclusions we have reached are certainly based on precarious reasoning.

Protagonist: Let's go on to consider how law might be helped by my proposal.

Antagonist: That's hardly likely.

Protagonist: Don't you think that the method of execution I advocate is better than those now in practice? Didn't you admit to that earlier?

Antagonist: I guess I did.

Protagonist: Is that not an advantage to the law? Would the proposal not impart a more beneficial aspect to the enforcement of capital punishment?

Antagonist: Before we can answer that question we must examine the reasons for the existence of the death penalty.

Protagonist: What do you think the purposes of capital punishment are? Why was it instituted?

Antagonist: The first and most obvious purpose must be exactly what its name implies: punishment for a capital crime.

Protagonist: And you consider death to be too drastic a punishment for a capital crime?

Antagonist: You know that very well from my earlier arguments.

Protagonist: What might be another reason for its existence?

Antagonist: The death penalty is certainly the most effective way of removing the criminal from society for all time. Furthermore, it saves the expense of maintaining him through a life sentence in prison or of rehabilitation in a mental institution.

Protagonst: Your first point is incontestable. Your second point, though, might be countered by a strong argument which has factual support; namely, that the expense involved in carrying out executions is substantial and, coupled with the maintainence of the pertinent facilities, adds up to an appreciable sum which might even match the cost of sustaining a man in prison.[3] I am sure you are aware of this consideration.

Antagonist: Yes. Still another purpose of the death penalty might be to dramatize the harsh fate in store for those who dare commit brutal or traitorous crimes.

Protagonist: In general the death penalty has no effective deterrent action. Those states which have abolished it have a capital-crime rate equal to or lower than the rate in those states which retain it. Furthermore, and this is even more astounding, certain studies have revealed the fact that there is a curious group of psychopaths who actually commit crimes in order to be executed. In other words, it is known that the death penalty can serve as an incentive to capital crimes.[4]

Antagonist: I am aware of that fact, which is a strong argument of the abolitionists. So far we have listed the retaliatory, protective, deterrent and financial reasons for the promulgation of the death penalty. I agree with you that the harshness of the penalty does not have much to do with actually deterring potential criminals, many of whom act in the heat of passion and uncontrollable emotions.

Protagonist: Perhaps the harshness of the punishment is its least important aspect. Nevertheless the concept itself should not be rejected solely on that basis, for that would be neglecting the other purposes for which it was brought into being. For after all, in this life one can rarely escape the idea of punishment.

Antagonist: But many capital crimes are committed by the mentally ill who cannot be held responsible for their actions.

Protagonist: Nevertheless, they must expect some form of punishment for what they have done. When a child is unreasonably mischievous, he is either punished or threatened with punishment, even though he, too, cannot be held ultimately responsible for his behavior. Misdeeds always connote punishment. As a child matures, extrinsically imposed measures help form the character and superego, which themselves gradually become major controlling forces embodying an appreciable capacity to punish.

Antagonist: I had never really conceived of the superego as a device for punishment.

Protagonist: But I am sure you can think of it as a reprimanding force. And reproof implies threat of punishment. There is not a controlling social force in human existence which is devoid of the idea of punishment.

Antagonist: Despite all this grandiloquence, I cannot subscribe to the notion that a mentally ill criminal must be executed.

Protagonist: Neither can I, in essence. What you are doing is making the idea of punishment paramount. I do not say that those who commit capital crimes should be executed primarily for punishment, nor even that they should be executed. The point I wish to make clear is that no matter how these men are handled, they must endure punishment or the threat of it in some degree.

Antagonist: If you continue along that course of reasoning, you will eventually undermine your own arguments. You will see that the death penalty is not a necessary means to that end.

Protagonist: Let me emphasize again that I am not arguing in support of the death penalty. Our task is to discuss its objectives and establish whether or not purposeful harshness and horror are indispensable adjuncts.

Antagonist: If it is to act as a deterrent or preventative, as you probably would say it is . . .

Protagonist: I didn't say that. In fact I agreed with you that it probably has little, if any, deterrent action.

Antagonist: Well, then, I say that these attributes are not indispensable.

Protagonist: Right. We are agreed that there are better ways to carry it out and that the method I advocate is one.

Antagonist: What has all this to do with the theme of this session?

Protagonist: We are discussing the relationship of the proposal to law, and we started out by trying to determine its detrimental aspect, if any. Now we're trying to see how it may be a boon to law. By introducing a form of execution which is humane and sensible, my proposal would endow law, itself a man-made thing, with another beneficent attribute and would impart to its offspring, capital punishment, more meaning than simply the crass aim of destroying a criminal life.

Antagonist: If you are saying that law engendered the death penalty out of a sincere concern for the good of mankind, and that this benevolent nature might be magnified twofold if it fostered a more humane, merciful death—a so-called "judicial euthanasia"—which at the same time enabled men to learn more about the human body, then I agree that your plan might be a boon to it. Of course, I feel that the concern which led to adoption of the death penalty was misguided; but I will pass up this point. Don't you feel that the introduction of mercy into the process of execution will destroy what little deterrent effect it has?

Protagonist: Perhaps so. But it will also destroy the incentive of those who use the death penalty as a form of suicide. I am sure that it is the thrill and notoriety attendant on a grotesque execution which appeal to these psychopaths. They would probably find nothing appealing in a merciful execution. So although one deterrent effect is lost, another is gained.

Antagonist: That assumption is reasonable enough. Let me now summarize my ideas. I believe that the introduction of your proposal would constitute serious tampering with the formality of law and would endanger the objectivity of justice. This to me is a consideration of tremendous magnitude. I believe furthermore that by introducing the idea of "judicial euthanasia" you do not enhance the beneficent nature of law as it now exists. Instead, you only enhance the appeal of capital punishment which itself is negative in theory and in results. Therefore, so far as law is concerned, I can see no convincing reason why the proposal should be endorsed.

Protagonist: And, of course, my ideas are directly contradictory to yours. In closing I would like to point out that even though capital punishment is somewhat negative, the introduction of the slightest degree of compassion in its practice would enhance the benevolence of the law which engendered it. I can see no detrimental effect of the proposal, and that is of utmost importance. Many of these points will undoubtedly be brought up for discussion again. Meanwhile let us turn our attention to how physicians and their research efforts might be affected if the proposal were to become a reality.

FIFTH SESSION

The Physician

Antagonist: Without a doubt most conscientious physicians will oppose the plan. After all, the primary aim of the profession is to aid mankind by alleviating pain and misery and by prolonging life. Ethically the physician is bound to the proposition that human life should never be taken.

Protagonist: In reality my plan does not entail the purposeful shortening of a human life. A condemned man is doomed by law to die. He cannot live. Any hope for his survival beyond the legally set date for execution is a hope for the breakdown of existing law. Socrates, too, could have escaped his fate; yet today he is among the most revered of men for having willingly submitted to execution after having so eloquently defended the justice of that fate. We have a deplorable tendency to take the importance of the distasteful aspects of law too lightly. We must face the fact that men must, by law, die. And if a physician can be instrumental in assuring a more merciful death, then that action is perfectly in line with the ideals of medical practice.

Antagonist: No matter how you try to explain it away, the physician, by experimenting on a criminal under anesthesia, directly involves himself in the premature termination of human life.

Protagonist: But you are putting the physician in the place of the executioner. His primary aim is not to end the man's life but to learn medical truths while at the same time mercifully implementing the law. If the man dies while the experiment is in progress, that is not in line with the physician's wishes. The longer the man lives, the more he will learn. As I stated before, the situation is analogous to a routine surgical operation in any hospital. The surgeon cannot be said to will the death of the patient, and if such a tragic accident occurs we do not for a moment think of branding him an executioner. The aim of a surgeon in any hospital would be exactly the same as that of researchers experimenting on a condemned man.

Now, if the condemned is still alive at the end of the experiment, he can be put to final death by an overdose of the anesthetic agent administered by a lay executioner specifically trained and employed for that purpose. Under these conditions how in the world can the physician be compared to an executioner?

Antagonist: But no matter what the physician's reasons are for becoming involved, by taking part he automatically becomes associated with the process of execution, and that makes him in part, at least, an executioner.

Protagonist: Let me try explaining it a different way. The point that causes me most concern is that executions today are a waste of human life. For the sake of argument I will go along with your objection about physicians being involved in the plan. Let us say instead that the entire setup is run by lay personnel; and that a well trained layman induces pentothal sleep and maintains subsequent anesthesia. Now, other highly trained laymen could very easily administer some new drug whose action had not before been tried on any human being, and could observe pertinent reactions. The resulting information would be of tremendous value. A physician is nowhere involved, but we still will have put the life of the condemned man to good use.

My only reason for suggesting that physicians perform the experiments is that they are most qualified to extract the greatest gain. If you insist that physicians remain aloof, I will counter with the proposal that lay persons assume the responsibility. In that case I must underscore the corresponding diminution in potential gain. The main point is still valid: executions as carried out today are an outrageous waste of human life; they could become a means for inestimable gain for human welfare. That is the end in view.

Antagonist: And I feel that physicians should not be the instruments of this gain.

Protagonist: I, of course, feel they should, because they are best suited. But I have shown that other means could be effectively used, without nullifying the worth of the proposal.

Antagonist: What possible gain could be immense enough to make all this discussion worthwhile? Don't you feel that we could learn just as much from animal studies? After all, in most instances of medical progress the initial discoveries were made on animals, and further elaborated on animals, before finally being translated into human terms. We had all the knowledge before it was applied to man.

Protagonist: That is true to a certain degree. But not all results of animal studies are valid for man. There are certain drugs which have a different effect, in fact an opposite effect, in dog and man. Furthermore, no matter how many times an experiment is tried on animals, to be meaningful to human existence it must be tried on man. The only thing I am trying to do is ensure that the initial human experiment will not jeopardize an innocent life.

Antagonist: Then wouldn't it be more reasonable to say that only those things already tried on animals be tried on condemned men?

Protagonist: Why is that more reasonable? If an idea is entirely new and must eventually be tried on a man, why not try it first on a human body which *must be destroyed by law?* Where is the immorality here?

Antagonist: You still have not answered my question regarding the value of the information to be gained.

Protagonist: Why do you insist on overlooking the chief difference between man and other forms of life? The human brain is the most highly developed of animal brains. The monkey or chimpanzee brain is the closest to it structurally. One of the best methods of studying brain structure is to create a small defect in the brain of a living animal, wait several days for a degenerative process to set in, and then kill the animal so that the degenerated tracts can be studied in specially stained serial sections of the brain. In this way the course of fiber bundles from one brain center to another can be traced. The data obtained are then applied to the analogous area of the human brain.

But the brains of men and animals are structurally not the same. Would it not be more reasonable to say that human brain anatomy should be learned from the human brain if suitable subjects are available for study? We would save millions of dollars and millions of man-hours of labor and have absolutely correct human data. I can state boldly that the first such human experiments would prove some current "truths" wrong and would reveal other undreamed-of things. Imagine that magnified a hundredfold!

Antagonist: Perhaps in that one respect human experimentation would be indispensable. But that is only a minor consideration. How about all the other significant studies which could conceivably be done on human volunteers who were not condemned? You are undoubtedly acquainted with the experiments involving new antimalarial drugs which were conducted on prisoner-volunteers during World War II. There were no drastic ill effects, and we did get the desired information.

Protagonist: That argument brings up two very important points, one practical, and the other moral. Let me take up the moral aspect first. Can you tell me the reason for allowing uncondemned prisoners to volunteer for certain experiments entailing a calculated risk?

Antagonist: That's an easy one to answer. Since the human risk has been previously minimized by animal tests, since human reactions must be known, and since the prisoners owe society a debt and can undertake this risk as partial repayment of it, what could be more logical than to allow them to do so?

Protagonist: Yes, it is an easy question to answer, and doesn't require profound insight. And your answer so far is logical. Now, would you say that the prisoners who volunteer do so out of a genuine desire to recompense the society they have wronged? Or, do the majority of them volunteer with the ultimate aim of gaining personal recognition and special considerations at parole hearings?

Antagonist: I am sure that some, in fact most, of them volunteer for the former reason—a sincere desire to repay society as best they can. Of course, the latter reason may motivate a few; but even so, the action benefits society.

Protagonist: But it's the ultimate motivation which counts. To me the latter reason is aimed at purely selfish ends and totally devoid of the characteristics of genuine repentance. In fact, this is being officially recognized in one of our states, now considering legislation which would automatically reduce the sentence of prisoners who volunteer as subjects for experiments of limited, scope and danger. I therefore must conclude that society, in allowing these men to literally "buy time" while at the same time refusing to allow the condemned man to donate his body without gain, is acting immorally. Plainly society needs the tests, and the men need their freedom. It's barter for mutually selfish ends. But now let's compare this situation with that of a condemned man. The latter has committed a capital crime, and owes society a great debt. Is that not so?

Antagonist: Yes.

Protagonist: And what can be his basic motivation for volunteering to die under experimentation, assuming that we allow him the choice?

Antagonist: Could it not be the same selfish motive you deplore?

Protagonist: How? The condemned *cannot* survive, for he is doomed by law.

Antagonist: He might decide to volunteer simply to avoid a harsh death. That is not a sublime reason.

Protagonist: But that is the *only* questionable aspect of his decision. All else would necessarily result from a desire to atone. Despite this inescapable conclusion, we persist in giving minor transgressors the chance to buy their way out, and refuse major wrongdoers a chance for partial redemption.

Antagonist: And that is your moral point?

Protagonist: Yes. It will come up again in the next session.

But now let me clarify the practical point I mentioned earlier. At present human experimentation is kept within limits which narrow down the amount of extractable knowledge. In the case of anti-malarial drugs animal experiments had in all likelihood furnished evidence beforehand that they were fairly safe. Any death would have simply been an unfortunate accident.

You know that some scientists were forced to experiment on themselves for want of volunteers. Pierre Curie used his own arm in studying radium burns. A few years ago the Nobel Prize in medicine was awarded to an obscure German who, as a surgical resident years before, passed a catheter through his own arm vein into his heart chambers, and thus took the first great step in the establishment of a modern clinical diagnostic procedure which has been indispensable in the advance of heart surgery. He had to submit himself to the test because there were no volunteers for such a new and apparently senseless experiment.

Now it seems to me that to execute many physically healthy men each year without at least giving such "senseless" ideas a try borders on the ridiculous. It is outright social immorality. I can see no good reason why this young and courageous resident had to risk his life to convince the world of the value of his idea, while we in turn wantonly destroy perfectly intact bodies for no tangible good. Could the heart of a condemned man under anesthesia not have been catheterized just as easily?

Antagonist: I am afraid I cannot argue your point.

Protagonist: Logic is hardly refutable. But there is still more to my practical point. Many educated people, physicians and non-physicians, have objected to my plan from the medical standpoint. Most of the former contend that the results of a solitary experiment are not valid in a scientific sense; that a series of studies is mandatory. I brought up the above example partly to show that the magnitude of a *single* human experiment can be enormous. A series of identical experiments is not necessary if conditions are well planned and the aims very profound. He who insists on such a series to validate his results displays a lack of imagination incommensurate with research talent, let alone genius. As I have already brought out, *just one* brain experiment would be invaluable. And a medical genius could conceivably find his way to tremendous new insights through a chain of independent human experiments.

Antagonist: You have clearly outlined the criticism of most antagonistic physicians, but on what practical grounds do non-physicians object?

Protagonist: Non-physicians, and a few physicians, too, maintain that all desired medical knowledge can be gotten from animals. Now most of these people are in no way connected with the health sciences, and if they are, not in the sense of being true basic research men. Yet they freely pass judgment. I am a physician, but it would be absurd for me to claim that I could say with any degree of justification what can and should be done, let alone *how*. I am sure that men now engaged in basic medical research could tell us how much a few such human experiments might advance medical science. Just imagine what Pasteur or Pavlov could have accomplished under such circumstances.

I have already mentioned how valuable the plan would be to neuroanatomy. There are many other examples. We are entering an era of whole organ transplants. I advocate that when any new whole organ transplant is to be tried, it be done first on a condemned man under anesthesia—if for no other reason than to clarify the technical details of the surgical manipulations involved. Long term results may still be feasibly obtainable in such a case.

The best way to achieve a successful transplant of human hearts would be to try it first on two living, healthy young men. And how are the first liver transplants to be done? Is the "new" liver to come from a freshly dead human body? It cannot be doubted that living bodies will offer the best possible chance for success. Far greater progress would have been made during the early years of needle biopsy techniques, and of heart, brain, and liver surgery if the procedures had been done for the first time on the strong bodies of doomed men instead of on the disease-ridden bodies of hopelessly ill patients.

Antagonist: Just as you criticize unqualified people for trying to pass judgment on the medical merits of your plan, are you not likewise out of line in trying to dabble in the legal problem of capital punishment and its merits? There seems to be an inconsistency on your part.

Protagonist: Not in the least. I only concern myself with the end results of the law, and evaluate them as does everyone else, by using my common sense. Our laws dictated that some men must die. Now plain common sense tells us that we do not use the most humane and profitable ways of putting a man to death. You and I have pretty much agreed on that. But when we turn our attention to a consideration of the potential medical progress my plan would afford, our evaluation requires more than common sense. It requires knowledge of current medical research and of the means needed to achieve the ends of this research. Even most practicing physicians are thus not qualified to pass judgment.

Let me summarize: The legal system which gave rise to capital punishment was based upon sociophilosophic factors. An understanding of these factors requires much formal training which you and I lack. However, the end result called capital punishment, and its actual implementation lie within the scope of our analysis.

No extraordinary training is necessary to evaluate present methods of execution by hanging, electrocution, the gas chamber, the guillotine, or firing squad. But a discussion of the medical merits of these methods, and of my plan, requires expert knowledge in the pertinent fields.

Antagonist: While what you say is true, in your zeal to underscore the magnitude of the good involved you may easily minimize ethical points of tremendous importance. Medical potentialities appear enormous only if taken by themselves; when they are counter-balanced against the great harm the plan might do, they lose much of their luster.

Even if I am not qualified to discuss medical considerations, my stand may still serve to represent all the factors which you so easily underestimate.

Protagonist: The subject of any debate should be dissected like a body, piece by piece. This session has dealt only with the medical aspects of the plan. The ethical and legal questions were dealt with previously and will be touched on again. If I appear to be overzealous in this regard, perhaps it is because the gains I anticipate stagger the imagination.

Antagonist: Because I am neither a physician nor a research man I cannot share your enthusiasm. I wonder if I would even if I were in such a position. It is clear that I have been at a disadvantage in the "dissection", as you put it, of this part of the general topic.

Protagonist: Perhaps you will be able to restore the balance in the next session, which will deal specifically with how the plan might affect society.

Antagonist: It will be delightful to return to common ground. I will feel satisfied if I can make you understand that the "bricks" we have been analyzing can be used to construct an edifice of such disharmony as to appall any man of sensibility.

SIXTH SESSION

The Public

Antagonist: The first big drawback so far as society is concerned is the amount of money needed to operate such a plan. Don't you think the cost would be prohibitive?

Protagonist: Undoubtedly large sums of money would be needed. But equally large sums of money are spent for research projects which would become superfluous if the sought-after information could be gained from the human body directly. So you see, my plan would require very little additional outlay of funds, if any.

Antagonist: But imagine the complex organizational problems the plan entails: committees at international, national, and state levels; and all the implied modifications of the penal system. Then there are the research facilities and teams, and transportation. All this adds up to quite a sum.

Protagonist: I refer you to my opening argument above. Also, the information to be gained from the operation of the plan would actually be invaluable. It isn't a matter of millions or billions of dollars, it's a matter of the knowledge to be gained. You cannot doubt that the results of human experimentation will be more meaningful than those of comparable animal studies. Even if it costs more the plan is still justifiable. The information thus "bought" would not be otherwise accessible in the remotely forseeable future.

Antagonist: Let's disregard these financial intricacies for a moment. I would like to point out that this type of scheme was tried, as part of the blackest, most barbaric chapter in the history of modern man.[6] Yet here you are, advocating that it be reinstituted in every civilized country on earth! Didn't the infamous Nazi crimes of World War II teach you the futility of such an endeavor?

Protagonist: "Reinstituted" is a poor word to use. What I am proposing has never before been tried in the *recorded* history of mankind. Let me ask you this: Were those crimes in Nazi Germany carried out during peacetime or wartime?

Antagonist: During World War II, of course

Protagonist: Now please recall my wording in the opening session—"by due process of civil law during peacetime." In essence that means under international law, and there you have the first great difference. There are many more. Can you tell me the legal basis used to condemn the victims of those crimes?

Antagonist: They were condemned under the laws of the Nazi regime.

Protagonist: Were those laws compatible with international standards?

Antagonist: No, definitely not.

Protagonist: Everyone knows that the victims were condemned to death on racial and political grounds. Consider this difference! And there are still others. Were the victims asked for consent before being experimented upon?

Antagonist: They were not, as far as I know.

Protagonist: Were the victims anesthetized before experimentation?

Antagonist: I must admit to ignorance of details, but I am fairly sure that most were not. In fact, that was one of the most barbaric aspects of the crimes.

Protagonist: Yes. The aims of most of the experiments were such as to necessitate consciousness on the part of the subject so that his subjective reactions might be indicated through speech. A few of the victims thus had to endure the most rigorous torture before fainting or dying. While we're on the topic, can you say what the aims of the experiments were?

Antagonist: I don't really know, but I have a notion that some of them were pretty silly.

Protagonist: Although some of the results could have been obtained from no other source than alive and conscious human beings, most of them were disgustingly superficial and were either already known or could have been obtained through more acceptable forms of research. The only really serious aims were of a military nature.

Now, another question: how would you characterize the scientists who carried out those crimes? Were they the world's most brilliant and benevolent researchers?

Antagonist: To be sure they were not. As I understand it they were unrestrained young men who were allowed to satisfy their sadistic urges because they were such fanatical servants of the party in power.

Protagonist: Did they represent the medical genius of Nazi Germany?

Antagonist: Most likely not.

Protagonist: The true medical genius remained in the large body of conservative German physicians, some of whom were downright shocked to learn of these experiments. Although they neither endorsed nor participated in the slaughter, their silence certainly leaves them open to criticism.

Antagonist: Have you now exhausted all differences? It is hardly conceivable that there could be more.

Protagonist: This may seem like gilding the lily, but there *is* one final consideration. The entire program of Nazi experimentation was carried out under the jurisdiction of a demented government guided by a senseless, barbaric philosophy. In the face of all this, how can you possibly compare what I propose to the Nazi crimes?

Antagonist: I will grant that there are significant differences in detail. But the quintessence of your proposal is very similar to that underlying those crimes.

Protagonist: What you really mean is that because the crimes involved human experimentation, the entire concept of extensive research on human subjects has become distasteful, and any proposal embodying that objective is automatically to be ignored.

In contradistinction to the Nazi plan, my plan involves condemnations imposed through civil law during peacetime. It is to be administered by a responsible international organization through supreme courts of nations and states. Experiments are to be carried out by scientists who demonstrate merit and rationality, as determined by a distinguished panel of medical researchers under the auspices of that international organization. Experiments are to be aimed at solving the riddles of human health and life. Finally, they will not be performed without the subject's consent, and every subject will be thoroughly anesthetized to ensure a painless death. My proposal is the antithesis of the Nazi plan.

Antagonist: I am fully aware of all these differences. Nevertheless, I find something repugnant in your proposal. It may be a manifestation of my emotional reaction to the Nazi crimes, but I cannot help believing that it has more substance than that.

Protagonist: Do you really believe that a thing once abused is always bad? In modern times, in fact during the last twenty-two centuries, we have had only one short period of direct experience with organized, sanctioned human experimentation; and that was in Nazi Germany. It was admittedly a nightmare. But human experimentation is not a bad thing simply because of that one abuse.

I think you will agree that religions in general are good for the welfare of mankind. In fact, they have underscored the growth and development of our culture. Yet the most indecent tortures have been inflicted in the name of religion. Countless wars have been fought, and millions of men mercilessly slaughtered through the abuse of religious principles. Despite this, religion itself has always emerged as glorious and exalted as ever. Then why should human experimentation, which can be so organized as to be perfectly in line with the mores of our civilization, be so abhorrent because of one instance of abuse? In the right hands and at the right time such abuse would be out of the question. Ours are the hands, and the time is ripe.

Antagonist: Pehaps I was a little presumptuous in my judgment. But I do think that the men involved in executing the plan would gradually develop a calloused attitude toward human life. They could very easily come to look upon the condemned man as mere protoplasm, to be used for their immediate interests and then discarded, instead of as the abode of a God-given soul.

Protagonist: It is my unshakable faith in the ability of men to execute this plan incorruptibly that compels me to advocate it so strongly. Could we not make such human experimentation a subspecialty of the medical profession? Accordingly, we might choose researchers of unquestionable scientific competence as guardians of the plan. They would first be given exhaustive training in law. These physician-lawyers then could be thoroughly imbued with the highest ideals of philosophy and religion. At the end they would emerge as physician-lawyer-philosopher-theologians who would be capable of extracting the maximum knowledge from studies on condemned men and at the same time be as incorruptible as is humanly possible. Only these men would be qualified to *conduct* the type of experiments in question although they might use plans submitted by other scientists.

Antagonist: Ideally your suggestions are superb, but it seems to me that if men were so trained, they would inevitably reach the conclusion that their actions were evil, that they were innocent instruments being used to rationalize a practice destined to foster insidious moral disintegration.

Protagonist: If you grant me that we *could* produce such superbly trained men to handle the actual experimentation, would that assure you sufficiently that corruption could be held in check?

Antagonist: Under those conditions, yes. But as I have maintained throughout this entire debate, your plan only tends to make the idea of capital punishment attractive. It makes a sort of martyr out of the condemned, and martyrdom is what I think should most be avoided, because it could be a big factor in lengthening the life of capital punishment.

Protagonist: That, too, is only speculation. Throughout recorded history capital punishment has been a part of human existence. I challenge you to cite authoritative proof to the contrary. My stand is based on history. Whether or not my proposal is adopted, the practice of capital punishment will persist, even in so-called enlightened nations, for many centuries. On what do you base your idea that capital punishment will eventually disappear?

Antagonist: On present trends. It seems to be disappearing already. It was very recently abolished in Brazil, and earlier in England.[7] In this country, several states have already dropped it, and several are in the process of doing so.

Protagonist: You mistake the fluctuations of popular opinion for an irreversible trend. England did drop it generally, but there are special cases today where it is still invoked, and a large part of the population is now clamoring for its general reinstatement. Complete abolition is rare.

Also, your idea that the abolitionists' cause is getting stronger is a false one. Before World War I only thirty-six of our states endorsed it. The hysteria and fear engendered by the war caused that number to be raised to forty-two. In the United States today, it is in use in forty states, although there are strong movements for its abolition in California, Ohio, Iowa, and in Massachusetts, where such a proposal was recently defeated three to one in a vote of the state legislature. Therefore you see that the trend is quite unpredictable and can suddenly reverse. Its direction at any specific time is dependent upon social, economic, and political factors which are for the most part unpredictable. Your stand is evidently based only upon hope.

Antagonist: Then you reject the idea that mankind will ever reach the degree of maturity needed to realize the uselessness and utter barbarity of the death penalty. I cannot share your pessimism. I have perfect confidence that it will ultimately be abolished. It may not be in our lifetime, or in this century, but it *will* happen eventually. I am against any action which would help to maintain the practice.

Protagonist: I appreciate your stand, but it seems to me much more precarious than mine which is based on history.

What would you say to a suggestion that the plan be instituted in only one state, which relies rather heavily on the death penalty, for a certain period of time, say a decade? After that time we could evaluate its effect, and see whether or not the death penalty in that state had become more popular. If it had come into more widespread use, I would be the first to say that my plan should be abolished. But at present we have absolutely no evidence for forming an opinion on this subject.

Antagonist: I grant you that we have no real facts. However, I am so thoroughly convinced that the plan would become corrupted and that it would perpetuate capital punishment that I am not willing even to try it on an experimental basis.

Protagonist: Even in view of the enormous medical benefits?

Antagonist: Even with those benefits in mind!

Protagonist: I can't help but feel that I represent the more righteous cause, since I am willing to undertake an experiment to settle this impasse. Experimentation is the only way to progress, even in the sphere of sociology. I challenge you to an impartial test to prove which of us is correct. I will construe any refusal on your part as tacit admission of insecurity.

Antagonist: You may construe my actions any way you wish! Under no circumstances will I take the risk of perpetuating capital punishment.

Protagonist: Let us leave this topic. Obviously we cannot agree.

We still need to discuss the possible good that society can do by fostering the plan. First, let me suggest that by doing so society would offer the condemned man a golden chance for restitution. After all, this is an inescapable aspect of capital punishment which we failed to touch upon in our earlier discussion. How can a man satisfactorily pay society simply by involuntarily losing his life?

Antagonist: That is a simple enough question to answer. In giving his life, he gives his dearest possession. That certainly is restitution enough.

Protagonist: But only in a very narrow sense. The man pays with his life, yes. It is a very dear price as far as he is concerned. But what does society gain? Payment implies the transfer of value. What is transferred from the condemned to society? Certainly not that abstract thing we call life? There is no transfer; there is only loss.

Antagonist: If your reasoning is right, it is only a further argument against the death penalty. There is neither deterrent effect nor the possibility of restitution. It should be done away with.

Protagonist: But there are many who feel that capital punishment is a good thing and should not be abolished, in fact, that it should be extended. That automatically calls for a little more thought on this aspect of restitution. As things now stand, there is no way to handle those convicted of capital crimes which allows them the opportunity to atone in any meaningful way. Now consider my plan. If society offers the condemned man the chance to reveal to us some of the most coveted secrets of nature, then it will have given him the chance to pay for his transgression. And he will pay not only the bare principal of a debt which he certainly owes, but interest, so to speak, a huge "tip" which promises far to surpass any real gain from the principal. I can conceive of no greater possibility for restitution from any known system of punishment, an undeniable transfer of something of value.

Antagonist: It is hard to deny that your plan might introduce the possibility of positive restitution.

Protagonist: It is a peculiar paradox that we spend millions of dollars in setting up experimental conditions involving ingenious arrays of glassware, makeshift apparatus, and all kinds of animals, yet, on the other hand, so callously and indiscriminately smash the magnificent experimental laboratory represented by the living body of the condemned man. What is even worse, we don't allow condemned human beings to die in as meaningful a way as that in which many condemned dogs die in our medical school laboratories.

Were I a condemned man, no matter how embittered, cynical, and contemptuous my outlook, I am sure that I could not help lamenting the totally empty means devised by society for punishing my wrongs. I would know deep within my soul that a death as outlined in my plan would be far more moral than a death in the gas chamber. I am sure that many other men now facing execution would agree with me. All I am trying to do is to allow them the opportunity to choose.

Antagonist: You are easily carried away by your own eloquence. But before you are totally blinded by the apparent "glory" of your plan, I would suggest that you take another look at the question of martyrdom. Don't you feel that if condemned men were allowed this choice, and if the majority did decide in favor of your proposed method, they would acquire an aura of saintliness? Would that not be defeating the purpose of capital punishment? Would it not extoll the transgressors?

Protagonist: Your objection has merit. I can answer only that the ultimate decision to experiment should be dependent upon judicial opinion. That is, some pertinent legal body should judge as to the suitability of the condemned man as a candidate for experimentation. No criminal, then, could be assured beforehand of the chance to die in this manner. The situation would always be in doubt, thereby preserving in each case what little deterrent effect there might be. Would you, as a prospective murderer, not think twice if you realized that the final decision would rest upon how you and the nature of your crime impressed the jury?

Antagonist: The uncertainty would be something of a deterrent, at least to me—assuming, of course, that I was not an irresponsible psychopath.

Protagonist: Yes, I think this modification provides an effective safeguard against endowing the transgressors with the essence of martyrdom which they surely do not deserve.

Now, there is another very important relationship between society and my plan, involving a key figure who is very easily forgotten. If a man is murdered, for what purpose does he die? If a child is kidnapped, slain, and brutally dismembered, for what purpose? Merely to snuff out the life of the killer brings to two the number of lives destroyed for no reason of any worth. Charles Starkweather killed eleven persons in Nebraska. For what purpose did they die? Why was Starkweather electrocuted? Did that action on the part of society restore the eleven victims?

Antagonist: It did not, and his execution had no real value in imparting significance to the death of his victims. I assume that you will now say that if Starkweather had been allowed to die as you advocate, some significance might have been imparted.

Protagonist: Yes, not only to the death of the eleven innocent victims, but also to his own. Some real value to mankind would have thereby resulted from the involuntary and unfortunate deaths of twelve persons. The degree of that significance does not enter into the situation. No matter how much or how little we might have learned from such an experiment, what really counts is the attempt to impart some *positive* meaning to capital punishment. The only meaning it has today is the negative one of permanently removing him from the offended society.

Objectively speaking, I cannot see where my stand is wrong. Of course it could be vehemently denounced on purely emotional grounds. Were a killer to feel extreme remorse and an uncontrollable desire to manifest repentance there would at present be no possible way for him to do so. Society has unconditionally precluded this possibility. And how do the families of the killers and their victims feel? Does electrocution lighten the physical and emotional burdens of the families concerned?

Antagonist: I sincerely doubt it. It would be absurd to think so.

Protagonist: If the killer were to die as I propose, would that lighten their burdens?

Antagonist: No more, I am sure. The plain fact is that the killer would be just as dead in either case, and I cannot see how the method of his death could make any appreciable difference.

Protagonist: The method isn't really the important thing. If we were to learn one new fact about human physiology in the process of his death, would that not make such a death more significant than one from which absolutely no knowledge was gained?

Antagonist: Yes, I suppose so. But you cannot make me admit that such a death would make the families feel better.

Protagonist: Whether they actually feel better about it or not is irrelevant. Will you at least agree that they would then have reason to feel better?

Antagonist: Logically speaking, yes.

Protagonist: So, you see, the basic significance of one's death is the crux of the matter. Granted society owes the condemned man no favors; it nevertheless stands to gain much by offering him a choice from which he, his victims, and their families too, will benefit.

Society must take stock of itself, in view of the paradoxes which have already been pointed out. What will be the judgment of our descendants regarding the way we now practice capital punishment in the light of how we reason it might best be handled?

Antagonist: Let me only say that if we discourse freely and thoroughly, as we are now doing, and think deeply and searchingly, as we all should try to do, and finally, if we decide wisely, as we all hope we can do, we need not fear the judgment of posterity.

SEVENTH SESSION

The Outlook

Antagonist: Just when did this idea of experimenting upon condemned men originate? It certainly must have been conceived before our time.

Protagonist: It was, long ago; but direct evidence has not survived. Medical histories by Galen and Celsus, indicate that the Hellenists of ancient Alexandria actually endorsed and practiced human vivisection. That would be about 300-200 B.C.

I first became aware of this through an obscure article[8] I found while probing into the history of the autopsy and dissection in general. The period of the Ptolemies was perhaps the most liberal age for the study of anatomy and for dissection of any kind in the history of civilized man. The subject has been treated delicately and rather superficially in the English and American literature, most authors inferring from the indirect evidence available to us that human vivisection was probably not practiced, at least on any significant scale, in the Alexandrian medical institutions of that time.

On the other hand, the reference I mentioned above probes into the matter a little more searchingly. From it emanates a rational inference that those ancient scientists probably had the benefit of a unique and well organized system of human dissection and vivisection. It seems that they, being true philosophers as well as scientists, were convinced that to know the human body as it actually exists one must of necessity practice vivisection.

Antagonist: Is there any way to prove whether or not men were vivisected at that time in the interests of science?

Protagonist: I am afraid not. Only indirect evidence is available.

Antagonist: Then it is strictly a matter of opinion. I personally cannot believe that such enlightened people could resort to such a thing for any reason.

Protagonist: But why did Galen and Celsus mention the practice? Surely they did not invent the concepts merely to make their historical works more interesting or entertaining. The plain fact that they did mention human vivisection is compelling evidence, which should not lightly be dismissed, that it was most likely known through practice. Their failure to emphasize it, as well as its disappearance from the literature of subsequent centuries, can easily be attributed to the disfavor into which the idea fell and has since persistently remained.

Antagonist: If that is so, then my ethical sense causes me to brand those philosopher-scientists as cruel barbarians.

Protagonist: You are hastily jumping to the conclusion that they had no knowledge of anesthesia in the modern sense. Do not forget that Alexandria at that time was the high point of civilization, having inherited the flower of Greek genius. It is consequently very difficult for me to believe that they did not have knowledge of anesthetic agents; abundant amounts of alcoholic beverages alone would be sufficient in some instances.

Antagonist: In view of the tenuousness of your evidence, I cannot conceive how any man, condemned or not, would have even considered such a fate at that time.

Protagonist: Your guess that condemned men were subjects of vivisection is correct. But consent was not involved. The Ptolemies stipulated that all condemned men were to be turned over to the researchers and to be used at their discretion. It was an involuntary form of execution, according to the reference I have quoted.

Their line of reasoning might have gone something like this: if a man is condemned by society, to protect itself and to punish the man, why should the procedure not be made more beneficial to mankind—even if the act seems repugnant? Such reasoning seemed so sound and logical that it compelled me to formulate the proposal at hand. Even the involuntary aspect is just. I introduced into my plan the condition of consent because it is more in keeping with our ideals of compassion.

Antagonist: It seems to me that any further discussion on points which have no factual basis would be ridiculous. Isn't there any period of history after Alexandria in which the topic again comes up?

Protagonist: Unfortunately not. It has never subsequently appeared in recorded history. Before formulating my proposal I searched many authoritative sources for any scrap of information on the subject. Inquiries at the Library of Congress, the Supreme Court, and the Justice Department (Medical Branch) in Washington, D. C., and at an internationally famous law school and library were dishearteningly fruitless. Furthermore, I have spoken to many American and foreign experts in law; but they could not direct me to a single example of serious debate or legislation on the matter. So, you see, this discussion of ours is the first dialectic exposition of an idea that has lain dormant for over 2000 years!

Antagonist: It is incredible that in our age, when everything conceivable appears in print, this rather simple idea should have escaped discussion.

Protagonist: A friend recently told me he had heard a report at a medical meeting by a researcher who a few years ago carried out electrocardiographic studies on a condemned man during the actual process of execution by hanging. The source of this information is reliable. Nevertheless, I have been unable to find any other reference to it or to ascertain whether or not the results were published. So, you see, the idea *has* occasionally been half-heartedly considered and even put into practice—albeit in a somewhat clandestine manner.

I deplore this hit-or-miss sort of thing. It is reminiscent of the old days of anatomy when competent and dedicated men were driven to body-snatching. The idea deserves more dignified treatment. Don't you agree that it's about time we gave it a thorough, open-minded appraisal?

Antagonist: I can see no harm in seriously discussing any idea; but endorsement for your plan is certainly out of the question as far as I am concerned.

Protagonist: Your admission that discussion would be healthful is victory enough for me. In the final analysis nothing else counts as much. I am not advocating, as a primary aim, that we adopt the plan. My first basic contention is that it be examined on a reasonable plane, unobscured by emotions and sentimentality.

Antagonist: And if it is rejected?

Protagonist: Under the conditions set forth who could doubt the sincerity of such action? As in propounding any other philosophic idea, one has only opinions and logic with which to argue. Facts are difficult to come by in these abstract realms.

Now, my second basic contention is less dogmatic than the first but equally sincere: One of the forty states in our nation now us-using the death penalty should introduce legislation allowing condemned men to *choose* this novel form of execution if they so desire. Should such an experiment, carried out for a specified length of time under the most stringent controls, fail to produce any real progress in medical research, or prove to make condemnations easier and more popular with juries, I will be the first to denounce the experiment, to stop it, and to recommend rejection of the plan for our time.

Antagonist: How can you be so sure that the condemned men would be inclined to go along with your plan? Aren't you basing a lot on mere opinion in that regard?

Protagonist: In anticipation of such criticism I decided to carry the question directly to a doomed man. Therefore, a little over a year ago I briefly interviewed a man who now faces electrocution. The interview was carried out in the presence of a prison official.

You can well imagine how difficult it is to talk to a man about his own impending death, but the conversation went off surprisingly well and with a seriousness of purpose which, I am sorry to say, has never been equaled in discussions with others less intimately concerned with the problem.

After emphasizing the purely hypothetical nature of my ideas, I asked the twenty-five-year-old doomed man which method he would prefer if the choice were offered him. His first reaction was one of apathy, and understandably so; for the concept of utility in death can hardly mean much to the one facing death.

After clarification of a few vague points, the man made a definite choice in favor of experimentation, rationalizing it at that time with the explanation that something learned from his body might be applied to maintain the health of his young daughter perhaps a decade or two hence. Imagine that—imagine the selfless consideration he gave to someone who would survive his own death.

I asked for and received written confirmation of that highly gratifying interview, in order to satisfy the skeptics.

Antagonist: Are you sure that his reasons were so noble, and that his main motivating impulses did not stem from a desire to avoid a harsh death?

Protagonist: Yes, I am convinced that they were noble. What else can we believe but that which he puts in writing? Here, see for yourself (figure 1). Note the quality of his reasons. Through a maze of misspellings and grammatical errors he has expounded as eloquently as could any philosopher the most cogent arguments in support of my plan.

Antagonist: The opinion of one condemned man does not necessarily speak for all condemned men. I have recently learned of similar interviews carried out by a prison official who was dubious of the merits of your plan. The condemned men he approached were firmly against the idea. Also, other uncondemned prisoners serving various sentences were interviewed and rejected the plan.

Protagonist: The results of my interviews with uncondemned

Dear Sir:

In responce to your request that I put my answer in writing here it is.

I feel the same today as I did yesterday when you asked me. I would gladly give you what you requested of me. And in doing so it might help others in many years to come and quite possiable even now.

It would also help me to think that I didn't succeed in making a total mess of my life, that I may have helped someone, somewhere, sometime.

I don't want you to think that I'm a brave man, or a hero, because that would be wrong, but if I must die, I must. but your way would be much more humane and at the same time beneficial to other's.

So I would like to apologize for the spelling, wording, writing of this letter. If your ever back down this way be sure to stop in, I enjoy talking to you.

Respectifuly Yours.

Figure 1.

Confirming a personal interview, this is a reproduction of an actual letter to the author from a condemned man who, at the time of this printing, is facing execution in one of our states.

prisoners are diametrically the opposite. I recently participated in such a study[9] involving men serving varying sentences for various crimes, men who professed violent opposition to the death penalty, in a state which is considering its abolition. Yet out of a total of 104 men who took the written test 89 supported my plan! Can you explain that away lightly?

All this shows that the results of the inquiries depend almost entirely on the way they are presented. It is analogous to asking permission to perform an autopsy after the death of a loved one. If the bereaved next of kin are approached tactlessly with an undercurrent of contempt for the end in view, of course permission will be refused. It is with compassion and understanding that one must approach those human beings on the receiving end of such a proposal. Had I spoken to the prisoners in the instance you cited earlier, I am sure the results would have been radically different.

In the last analysis, all that matters to me is that one condemned man definitely endorses my plan. If only one out of every ten doomed men chose it, the plan would certainly deserve implementation. In that case, of the almost 3,500 persons executed under civil law since 1930 in the United States alone, 350 could have given us the opportunity to blaze new trails into the darkness of medical ignorance. How much more would we now have known, and how many more persons would have lived longer and happier lives?

That loss is incalculable in terms of any conventional standard of values. But the continuity of that loss can be stopped. At presend 50 to 60 men are executed in the United States annually. If only one out of ten preferred to undergo research (and I am sure that many more than that would), we could salvage knowledge of inestimable value from what would otherwise be atrocious waste.

Antagonist: There is an immense amount of food for thought in those comments. I wonder what most of the condemned men now in death houses throughout the country might say of the plan. There is much room for further research in that regard.

Protagonist: It is regrettable that one must start from the bottom in that research, as you call it. What I want to do is stimulate thought and discussion among the sensible and intelligent, law-abiding citizens who constitute the enlightened of our society. Why should we start with the condemned and the imprisoned in probing the merits of this idea? We should instead discuss it thoroughly among ourselves and decide first among ourselves, disregarding the viewpoints of those who have forfeited their right to speak about how we might conduct the affairs of our civilization.

FOOTNOTES

1. J. Kevorkian, "Capital punishment or capital gain? A proposal for execution of condemned prisoners through anesthesia for medical experimentation." Controversial Issues in Twentieth Century Criminology, New York: Philosophical Library, (in press).
2. J. D. Nicola, "The case against the Death Penalty," Information, June, 1959 (Reprint).
3. Ibid.
4. H. J. Klare, "Hanging the Sick," New Statesman & Nation, XLVI (August 1, 1953) 130-131.
5. A. C. Ivy, "The history and ethics of the use of human subjects in medical experiments," Science, CVIII (July 2, 1948) 1-5.
6. A. Mitscherlich, and F. Mielke, Doctors of Infamy (New York: Henry Schuman, 1949).
7. G. Playfair, and D. Sington, "A challenge to abolitionists," New Statesman & Nation, LII (July 21, 1956) 63-64.
8. L. Edelstein, "Die Geschichte der Sektion in der Antike," Quellen und Studien zur Geschichte der Naturwissenschaften und der Medizin, III, no. 2, (Berlin: Springer-Verlag, 1932) 50-106.
9. W. A. Lunden, and J. Kevorkian, to be published.